Intermittent Fasting

The Ultimate Guide For Losing Weight And Staying Healthy For Life and achieve Rapid Weight Loss

(Living a Healthy Lifestyle and Increase Energy While Eating the Foods You like)

Keith Love

Published by Jason Thawne Publishing House

© Keith Love

Intermittent Fasting: The Ultimate Guide For Losing Weight And Staying Healthy For Life and achieve Rapid Weight Loss

(Living a Healthy Lifestyle and Increase Energy While Eating the Foods You like)

All Rights Reserved

ISBN 978-1-989749-50-0

This document is geared towards providing exact and reliable information in regards to the topic and issue covered. The publication is sold with the idea that the publisher isn't required to render accounting, officially permitted, or otherwise, qualified services. If advice is necessary, legal or even professional, a practiced individual in the profession should be ordered.

- From a Declaration of Principles which was accepted and approved equally by a Committee of the American Bar Association and a Committee of Publishers and Associations.

In no way is it legal to reproduce, duplicate, or even transmit any part of this document in either electronic means or in printed format. Recording of this publication is strictly prohibited and any storage of this document isn't allowed unless with proper written permission from the publisher. All rights reserved.

The information provided herein is stated to be truthful and consistent, in that any liability, in terms of inattention or otherwise, by any usage or abuse of any policies, processes, or directions contained within is the solitary and also utter responsibility of the recipient reader. Under no circumstances will any legal responsibility or blame be held against the publisher for any reparation, damages, or monetary loss due to the information herein, either directly or indirectly.

Respective authors own all copyrights not held by the publisher.

The information herein is offered for just informational purposes solely, and is universal as so. The presentation of the information is without contract or any type of guarantee assurance.

The trademarks that are used are without any consent, and also the publication of the trademark is without permission or backing by the trademark owner. All trademarks and brands within this book are for clarifying purposes only and are the owned by the owners themselves, not affiliated with this document.

TABLE OF CONTENTS

PART 1 1

INTRODUCTION 1

CHAPTER 1: BRIEF INTRODUCTION ON FASTING IN GENERAL 3

CHAPTER 2: WEIGHT GAIN AND WEIGHT LOSS 7

CHAPTER 3: A MORE DETAILED INTRODUCTION TO INTERMITTENT FASTING AND HOW IT WORKS 10

CHAPTER 4: BREAKING MYTHS THAT SURROUND INTERMITTENT FASTING 21

CHAPTER 5: THE BENEFITS OF INTERMITTENT FASTING ... 23

CHAPTER 6: DIET EXAMPLES AND RECIPES 26

1. SALMON AND TABBOULEH BOWL 30

2. PORK CHOPS WITH HOLLANDAISE AND ASPARAGUS .. 32

3. CHEESE AND TOMATO OMELET 34

4. FRIDGE SALAD 35

5. TIGER PRAWN CURRY WITH BASMATI RICE 36

6. CREAMY GARLIC MUSHROOM AND TOAST 38

7. SMOKED SALMON PITA PIZZA 39

8. HERB AND SPICE CRUSTED BAKED CHICKEN BREASTS .. 40

9. KETO CHEESEBURGER 41

FOR THE BURGER PATTIES: 41

CHAPTER 7: HOW TO GRADUALLY TRANSITION TO INTERMITTENT FASTING 44

CHAPTER 8: HOW TO SUCCEED – EFFECTIVE TIPS AND TRICKS AND HACKS 48

CONCLUSION.. 51

PART 2.. 53

BREAKFAST... 72

POACHED EGGS WITH MUSHROOMS: 135 CALORIES 72

QUICK BRUSCHETTA: 204 CALORIES 74

CAULIFLOWER BAKE: 157 CALORIES 75

APPLE AND WALNUT PORRIDGE: 159 CALORIES.............. 76

ASPARAGUS OMELETTE: 100 CALORIES........................... 77

STIR FRY BOK CHOY: 236 CALORIES 78

APPLE AND CUCUMBER REFRESHER: 60 CALORIES 80

SWEET AND SAVOURY SALAD: 240 CALORIES.................. 81

CHEESE & ONION FRITTATA: 195 CALORIES..................... 82

FRUITY OATBARS: 135 CALORIES IN 1 BAR 83

FRESH FRUIT SALAD: 175 CALORIES................................. 85

SCRAMBLED EGG WITH CHIVES: 190 CALORIES 86

HOT GRAIN BREAKFAST: 188 CALORIES........................... 87

FRUIT & GINGER SMOOTHIE: 128 CALORIES.................... 88

SPINACH & ONION OMELETTE: 184 CALORIES................. 89

OATMEAL & BLUEBERRY BREAKFAST: 95 CALORIES 90

- MISO AUBERGINES: 153 CALORIES 91
- LEMON AND PARSLEY COUSCOUS: 249 CALORIES 93
- CARROT AND MANGO CRUSH: 185 CALORIES 94
- SPICY ONION & TOMATO SALAD: 47 CALORIES 95
- FETA TORTILLA WRAP: 267 CALORIES.............................. 96
- SPICED FRUIT SMOOTHIE: 192 CALORIES.......................... 97
- TOMATOES WITH OKRA & ONION: 71 CALORIES............. 98
- VEGETABLE BROTH: 236 CALORIES 99
- BLUEBERRY-PACKED SMOOTHIE: 160 CALORIES............ 100
- EDAMAME SALAD: 127 CALORIES 101
- CHINESE GINGER VEGETABLES: 213 CALORIES............... 102
- BLUEBERRY QUARK PANCAKE: 130 CALORIES 104
- FRESH MEDITERRANEAN SALAD: 132 CALORIES............ 105
- CARROT & LENTIL SOUP: 237 CALORIES 107
- ORANGE FRUIT SALAD: 120 CALORIES............................ 108
- RED PEPPER SOUP: 77 CALORIES 109
- STUFFED PEPPER: 303 CALORIES 109
- SPICED FRUIT SALAD: 70 CALORIES................................ 111
- SUMMER SALAD: 83 CALORIES....................................... 112
- TWIRLY PASTA WITH TOMATOES, SPINACH & CHEESE: 339 CALORIES 113
- PEANUT BUTTER AND FRUIT WAFFLE: 165 CALORIES 114

- SPICY CAULIFLOWER: 140 CALORIES 115
- BASIL & TOMATO SCRAMBLED EGGS: 195 CALORIES 116
- BAKED SPICED GRAPEFRUIT: 62 CALORIES 117
- MEDITERRANEAN VEGETABLE ROAST: 91 CALORIES 118
- SPAGHETTI WITH COURGETTE (ZUCCHINI) & ONION: 342 CALORIES 119
- SPICED ORANGES: 100 CALORIES..................................... 120
- CAULIFLOWER SOUP: 87 CALORIES 121
- MIXED ROAST VEGETABLES WITH PASTA: 313 CALORIES 123
- CHEESY TOASTY BREAKFAST: 99 CALORIES..................... 124
- SWEET & SOUR SALAD: 87 CALORIES............................... 125
- VEGETABLE GOULASH: 313 CALORIES.............................. 126
- PEAR AND GINGER SMOOTHIE: 190 CALORIES 127
- COLESLAW: 79 CALORIES... 128
- CHINESE GINGER VEGETABLES: 225 CALORIES............... 129
- CUCUMBER, MINT & ORANGE REFRESHER: 105 CALORIES 131
- QUICK MINESTRONE SOUP: 197 CALORIES..................... 132
- PASTA WITH TOMATO SAUCE: 190 CALORIES................ 133
- FRESH FRUIT AND VEGETABLE JUICE: 145 CALORIES...... 135
- CARROT AND CUMIN SOUP: 108 CALORIES 135
- TOFU AND QUINOA: 240 CALORIES................................ 137

SPICY APPLE AND KIWI SMOOTHIE: 80 CALORIES 138

YOGHURT WALDORF SALAD: 233 CALORIES 139

SPICED LENTIL STEW: 187 CALORIES 140

CONCLUSION 142

ABOUT THE AUTHOR 142

Part 1

Introduction

This book entitled is all about dieting, fasting, and maintaining a healthy lifestyle. It contains proven steps and strategies on how to lose weight, increase your energy and mental focus, as well as improve your overall health through intermittent fasting.

All throughout the history of time, fasting has been a means for healthy reform, prayerful contemplation, reflection, and protest. It is actually defined as the abstinence from various foods and drinks, especially for religious, experimental, or medical purposes.

Religious groups are especially inclined to fasting. They do it individually or as a community. The famous Mahatma Ghandi once fasted for twenty-one days as a protest to the British rule in India.

Today, intermittent fasting is done to cleanse the body as well as achieve other benefits, such as weight loss, diabetes treatment, and heart disease prevention. Fasting restricts the short term storage of energy. Hence, it taps into the fat reserves of the body and promotes weight loss and metabolism. It also contributes to numerous health benefits.

In this book, you will learn more about intermittent fasting. You will learn about the recipes and meal plans you can follow to incorporate this diet into your day to day life. You will also learn how to transition from your normal eating routine into this diet.

Thanks again for downloading this book, I hope you enjoy it!

Chapter 1: Brief Introduction on Fasting In General

Food is a primary necessity. You need to eat food in order to survive and function properly. When your body does not get enough nutrients, you become at risk of various diseases and you lack energy to do your tasks.

However, not eating for a certain amount of time can also be good for you. When you fast, you hold yourself from food. You abstain for a definite timeframe. This practice is not entirely new. In fact, it has been around for thousands of years. People from different cultures and religions practice fasting.

Fasting is only recommended to people who are healthy. Those who are malnourished, underweight, or have pre-existing medical issues should consult their doctor before fasting. Likewise, those who have recently gone through a surgical procedure should avoid fasting.

When you fast, your body enters into a self-preservation state to counter starvation. It begins to increase your cortisol production and slows down your metabolism. Cortisol is a type of stress hormone. When you are stressed, your body releases more cortisol. This is not healthy because too much cortisol can exhaust you mentally and physically.

When you fast longer than necessary, you damage your muscles. This decreases your chance of losing weight. Muscles are vital for burning excess fat. Your cortisol also releases acids from your muscles and converts them into sugar. Then, this sugar is brought to your brain, kidneys, and red blood cells. The human brain instantaneously uses sugar as fuel, even though it can use fat.

Also, when you fast for too long, you increase your chances of craving for food and gaining back the weight that you lost. Likewise, your body releases less thyroid hormones. If your body does not have enough thyroid hormones and muscle tissues, your metabolism suffers.

When you fast for too long, you also deplete your sources of nutrients, such as vitamins, minerals, carbohydrates, proteins, and fatty acids. You become prone to experiencing headaches, fatigue, dehydration, constipation, anemia, hypoglycemia, and muscle weakness.

Thus, you should only fast for the necessary periods of time. For example, if you want to lose weight, you can fast for twenty-four hours. It is not recommended to fast for as long as thirty-six hours because it can be dangerous to your health.

In addition, you should avoid performing any strenuous physical exercises when you fast. You can perform light exercises, such as walking and jogging. You should also avoid operating heavy machinery.

See to it that you drink sufficient amounts of water to keep your body hydrated. You can also consume soups and fruits. Avoid eating anything that is not nutritious. Consult a dietician to find out what is best for your body.

Chapter 2: Weight Gain and Weight Loss

Intermittent fasting can affect your hormones. Before you go through this diet, you have to understand that body fat is your body's way of storing energy. If you do not eat anything, your body changes certain things to make your stored energy easier to access.

Your insulin, human growth hormone, and norepinephrine are all affected when you fast. Insulin usually increases when you eat. So, when you fast, your insulin levels go down and promote fat burning. Conversely, your HGH levels may increase when you fast. This hormone is responsible for your muscle gain and fat loss. Also, your norepinephrine breaks down your body fat into free fatty acids that may be burned for energy.

Weight Loss with Intermittent Fasting

Most of the people who embark on intermittent fasting aim to lose weight. This diet works for them because it encourages them to consume fewer calories. In a review study done in 2014, it was found that intermittent fasting may result in weight loss. In fact, it can reduce body weight by three to eight percent in just three to twenty-four weeks.

In addition, the researchers have found that people on this diet can lose 0.25 kg each week. They can also lose four to seven percent of their waist circumference or belly fat.

Weight Gain with Intermittent Fasting

Then again, intermittent fasting may also lead to weight gain. Americans are particularly known for consuming more calories than necessary. This is the main reason why a lot of them are obese and diabetic. They are also at risk of heart diseases and other chronic illnesses.

Intermittent fasting ultimately translates to the intake of fewer calories over a certain amount of time. Thus, it makes sense that an individual who typically fasts also eats less unhealthy fats, processed foods, and refined sugar throughout this timeframe.

However, if you are not disciplined enough, you may go back to your old eating habits. Even worse, you may consume more calories than the normal because you feel that you have been deprived of food. This is the main reason why intermittent fasting does not work on some people. They simply lack the discipline to follow through.

Chapter 3: A More Detailed Introduction to Intermittent Fasting and How It Works

Intermittent fasting occurs between periods of fasting and non-fasting. It is about taking intermittent fasting schedules that you have to stick with. It is also similar to caloric restriction, which is another form of dietary restriction or dietary energy restriction.

When you embark on this diet, you allow your body to function differently whenever you eat and do not eat. With intermittent fasting, you are required to eat for extended periods of time. You also have to eat what you have to eat for the entire day on your pre-determined feeding windows.

For instance, you may fast for sixteen hours today and then eight during the next eight hours. If you prefer to fast on a daily basis, you can fast for twenty hours and then eat during a four-hour window. In addition, you may eat for the whole day but fast the following day.

You may try different variations of this diet. In fact, it is recommended that you try as many diets as you can until you find one that is suitable for your needs and preferences. Once you find the one that works best, you have to stick with it.

Different Types of Intermittent Fasting

Daily Fasting

This type of fasting is also known as the Leangains model. It was developed by Martin Berkhan and it is about fasting for sixteen hours and having an eight-hour eating period.

When you do a daily fast, you have to skip breakfast and another meal. Basically, you should only eat one meal per day. However, you still need to ensure that you receive all the calories your body needs.

Weekly Fasting

This is done once a week. Do not worry because not eating for twenty-four hours is not dangerous, unless you have an existing medical condition. Consult your doctor before you embark on this diet.

When you do a weekly fast, you should remove two meals from your diet every week. For example, you can eat at 12 PM today and not eat anything until 12 PM tomorrow.

Alternate Day Fasting or Every Other Day Feeding/Fasting

It is about fasting for twenty-four hours and then not fasting for the next twenty-four hours. Since it involves restricting caloric intake on alternating days, it may help prolong your life span.

Modified Fasting

It is about limiting your caloric intake during your fasting days. You should not mistake it for prohibiting any calories. You may allow yourself to consume twenty percent of your usual caloric intake, for example. Make sure that you discipline yourself and not go beyond this limit.

According to researchers, modified fasting is the most effective of all types of intermittent fasting.

Short Intermittent Fasting

Experts recommend doing this type of fasting every day or three times a week. Just make sure that you have a condensed feeding window. For example, you may consume calories during a six-hour or eight-hour feeding window before fasting.

See to it that you also consider other factors, such as your physical activities, caloric needs, food choices, and recovery period when you fast. You also need a consistent schedule.

Most dieters actually prefer short intermittent fasting to long intermittent fasting. Short intermittent fasting focuses on choosing healthy foods and refraining from eating snacks and desserts.

This type of diet is ideal for those who are aiming to shed a few pounds or tone their body. It is also ideal for people with health problems, such as blood sugar and metabolic issues.

Then again, short intermittent fasting is not ideal for those who consume very few calories as well as those whose bodies need plenty of calories. For example, if you are an athlete and you are very active, this diet may not work for you since you need to consume plenty of calories to stay in top shape.

Long Intermittent Fasting

It should be done one to two times a week. It should also last for twenty-four hours. So, if you embark on this diet, you have to wait for twenty-four hours before you eat again.

For example, if you stopped eating at 1 PM on a Monday, you can only eat again at 1 PM the following Tuesday. This type of diet ensures that your body receives the calories it needs to continue functioning properly. It also allows your body to undergo deep cellular cleaning.

Keep in mind that long intermittent fasting is not similar to a crash diet. Crash diets are dangerous and not recommended by experts. These kinds of diets deprive the body the calories it needs to function normally. Long intermittent fasting is about self-control. Each time you crave for food, you need to control yourself. Make sure that you do not binge when you get hungry.

Notes on Intermittent Fasting

If you have a weak body or you are prone to stress, embarking on intermittent fasting is not advisable. It may be too stressful for you in the long run. Likewise, it is not advisable for individuals suffering from metabolic and blood sugar problems. It is also not ideal for physically active people who need to consume a lot of calories.

Nonetheless, if you have a healthy body, you can go through intermittent fasting without putting yourself at risk of diseases. You can skip breakfast and still be able to go through your day normally. However, you need to drink sufficient amounts of water throughout the day, as well as three hours before your bedtime.

While on this diet, you also need to eat lean proteins. Experts recommend restricting your feeding window to eight hours each day. Refrain from consuming carbohydrates, especially if you are trying to lose weight. Bread, pasta, and potatoes should be avoided.

Load up on healthy fats, such as eggs, avocados, olive oil, nuts, and coconut oil. These foods can help your body transition to the fat-burning mode from the carbohydrate-burning mode. Once you reach this mode, you will no longer crave for unhealthy foods. So, if you used to eat lots of junk food, sugary snacks, and processed foods, you will not miss them anymore. You will also feel less hungry throughout the day. Even better, your metabolism will improve.

Just like with any other diet, you should not expect instant results. Intermittent fasting can take a while to have effects on your body. You may have to wait for a few days or weeks to adjust to this diet. As a beginner, you may experience discomfort during the first few days. However, as you get used to intermittent fasting, you will find it easier to restrict your calorie consumption as well as not get hungry even after eighteen hours of not eating anything.

Intermittent fasting is also good for your gut. It supports the growth of healthy bacteria in your body. It also improves your immune system. With a healthy immune system, you will be able to sleep and concentrate better. You will also have more energy levels as well as better mental clarity.

The Effects of Intermittent Fasting on Men and Women

Researchers have found that intermittent fasting has different effects on men and women due to the differences between their bodies. Men, for example, are able to burn fat faster than women. Women tend to store more fat than men. Men also tend to aim for muscle building while women tend to aim for weight loss.

Intermittent fasting is also effective in improving men's insulin sensitivity. However, it may not have the same effects on women. Nonetheless, intermittent fasting also reduces women's triglycerides and improves their HDL while it reduces men's triglycerides yet maintains their HDL.

Both men and women who are obese can lose weight through intermittent fasting. This diet can help them burn fat as well as reduce their levels of blood pressure, LDL cholesterol, total cholesterol, and triglycerides. Then again, women at their reproductive and pre-menopausal stages may get different results.

Intermittent fasting is great if you are trying to lose weight since it requires a strict calorie count. So, if you do not eat for sixteen hours, your body lowers its calories and loses weight faster.

Intermittent fasting is also effective in promoting a healthy lifestyle. You really have to exert effort in preparing and cooking your meals since you are not allowed to eat processed goods, fast food take-outs, and other unhealthy food choices.

Since you are fasting, you also no longer have to worry about eating every few hours. You do not even have to have a complicated schedule. You can just skip one to two meals per day.

The Science Behind Intermittent Fasting

There have been plenty of studies with regard to the benefits and risks of fasting. However, these studies have only considered animal models. They have found that intermittent fasting can be beneficial to people with diabetes, heart diseases, neurological disorders, and cancers. On the other hand, studies on humans have found that intermittent fasting can lead to weight loss, blood sugar control, and cholesterol reduction.

Chapter 4: Breaking Myths that Surround Intermittent Fasting

Intermittent fasting is practiced by a lot of people. Surprisingly, however, many people still have misconceptions about this diet. The following are some of the common myths that surround it:

Intermittent fasting is merely a fad diet.

No, intermittent fasting is a proven method for achieving weight loss and other health benefits. It is not the same as a detox either.

Intermittent fasting makes you lose muscle.

No, you will not lose muscle while on this diet. You can skip eating protein for several hours and still retain your muscle. Do not worry because your body will not break down its protein reserves if you stop eating for a while. Take note that the human body is capable of preserving muscle even at a fasted state.

Intermittent fasting makes your body go into starvation mode.

No, your body will continue burning calories while you are on this diet. Then again, researchers have found that the metabolic rate does not get affected until seventy-two to ninety-six hours have gone by. When you fast for a short while, you give your metabolic rate a chance to increase.

Intermittent fasting is the same for every person.

No, intermittent fasting is different for men and women. It is different for people with different lifestyles, weight, body mass index, etc. So, if you have a friend who embarks on intermittent fasting, his results may not exactly be the same as yours.

Chapter 5: The Benefits of Intermittent Fasting

Intermittent fasting can result in fat loss, which is great if you want to get fitter. However, that is not the only benefit you can get from this diet.

Intermittent fasting can also make your lifestyle simpler.

Who doesn't want a life that is simple and stress-free? With intermittent fasting, you no longer have to worry about when you have to eat. You can simply skip breakfast and go about your day. You can also skip lunch and then eat dinner. The premise of this diet is cutting out one or two meals from your day.

With this being said, you also get to prepare and cook one to two less meals. You can have more time to do other things or relax yourself. What's more, you can save money.

Intermittent fasting can also help you live longer.

According to experts, restricting your caloric consumption can help strengthen your body. This actually makes sense because when you starve yourself, your body automatically adjusts to the situation and finds ways to survive.

When you fast, you sort of starve yourself; but not to the extent of harming your health. You simply cut a meal or two from your diet in order to make your body burn fats.

Intermittent fasting can also reduce your risk of cancers.

Researchers have found that intermittent fasting is also helpful to people who have cancers. In a study of ten cancer patients, it was found that fasting can reduce the side effects of chemotherapy. In a similar study, it was found that alternate day fasting can help cancer patients increase their survival rate.

Intermittent fasting is a lot easier than dieting.

Diets tend to fail because dieters do not stick with them. They do not have enough discipline and determination to follow through. With intermittent fasting, you can easily achieve your target results.

In a study of obese individuals, it was found that the participants were able to quickly adapt to their intermittent fasting routine. Unlike other diets, such as the low carb diet, you do not have to keep thinking about the foods that you are not allowed to eat. You can still eat your usual foods, but you have to watch your caloric intake.

In addition, you can easily remember not to eat for twenty-four hours. While you may feel a little bit of discomfort at first, you will surely get used to your new routine quickly. You will no longer feel hungry and you will be able to get over the idea of not eating anything for a certain period of time.

Chapter 6: Diet Examples and Recipes

Intermittent fasting is simple and straightforward. You skip certain meals and reap the benefits of your diet. Then again, even though you can skip meals, you should still ensure that you get all the nutrients your body needs. You also need to make sure that you consume the right amount of calories every day.

What can you eat while on intermittent fasting? During your non-fasting days, you can indulge a little and go for a slice of pizza or a cup of ice cream. There is no need to turn your back on your favorite snacks and desserts. You can still eat your favorite foods. Just make sure that you control yourself and do not fall back to your old eating patterns.

During your fasting days, you can have snacks between your meals to help you stay satiated. During days when the weather is hot, you can eat fruits and light meals. If you are not a big fan of fruits, vegetables, lean meats, and whole grains, you can add tasty dressings and seasonings to your meals. This way, you can satisfy your taste buds and still eat healthy.

Furthermore, you can experiment with various recipes. Going on intermittent fasting should not make your life boring. If you have no idea on where to begin, here is a sample menu you can try for the week:

Monday
Breakfast:
1 scrambled egg
1 ounce smoked salmon
1 cup of black coffee

Snack:
½ banana

Lunch:

½ English muffin with 1 tablespoon tomato sauce and 1 tablespoon low-fat mozzarella

Snack:
½ banana

Dinner:
1 plate of feta salad
1 bowl of butternut squash soup

Tuesday
Breakfast:
½ cup raspberries
¼ cantaloupe
1 glass of water

Snack:
1 bowl of miso soup

Lunch:
1 bowl of tossed salad that consists of 1 cup of chopped lettuce, 10 shrimps, ½ cup

chopped cucumber, and 1 tablespoon ranch dressing

Snack:
1 turkey wrap

Dinner:
1 poached egg
6 steamed asparagus spears
½ English muffin

Wednesday
Breakfast:
½ cup raspberries
1 cup of black coffee

Snack:
10 pieces of pistachio nuts

Lunch:
1 bowl of tossed salad that consists of 3 cups of mixed greens, ½ boiled egg, 1

tablespoon low-calorie dressing, and 2 tablespoons grated parmesan cheese

Snack:

7 pieces of almond nuts

Dinner:

1 bowl of tossed salad that consists of 3 cups of mixed greens, ½ boiled egg, 1 tablespoon low-calorie dressing, ½ cantaloupe, and 3 ounces smoked salmon

Recipes for Intermittent Fasting

Here are sample recipes you can try:

1. Salmon and Tabbouleh Bowl

Ingredients:

- 300 grams of salmon fillet
- 1 tablespoon of olive oil
- black pepper
- salt

- 240 grams of cauliflower
- 35 grams of red cabbage (shredded)
- 25 grams of sugar snap peas (chopped)
- 50 grams of red pepper (chopped)
- 15 grams of red onion (sliced)
- 15 grams of parsley (chopped)
- 2 tablespoons of chopped mint
- 75 grams of crumbled feta
- 3 tablespoons of olive oil
- 2 teaspoons of lemon juice

For the basil yogurt dressing:
- 1 teaspoon of lemon juice
- 1 tablespoon of basil (chopped)
- 1 tablespoon of full fat Greek yogurt
- black pepper
- salt

Instructions:

Preheat your oven to 180°C and line your baking tray with greaseproof paper. Then, season your salmon with pepper, salt, and olive oil. Roast it in the oven for twenty-five minutes or until the skin becomes crispy.

Place the cauliflower in your food processor and process it until it has a rice consistency. Put it in a bowl. Microwave it for four minutes and then let it cool. In a separate bowl, combine olive oil, pepper, salt, and lemon juice. Add the red cabbage, red onion, sugar snap peas, red pepper, and fresh herbs. Add the dressing and some of the feta to your cauliflower rice. Toss everything.

In another bowl, mix the basil yogurt dressing. Put the tabbouleh in a serving container. Top with the rest of the feta, basil yogurt dressing, and roast salmon.

2. Pork Chops with Hollandaise and Asparagus

Ingredients:
- ½ cup of butter

- 3 egg yolks
- 3 pork loin chops
- 1 tablespoon of lemon juice
- 2 tablespoons of lard
- 300 grams of asparagus spears
- pepper
- salt

Instructions:

Prepare the Hollandaise. Put the butter in a large jar. Melt it inside your microwave. Add the lemon juice and egg yolks. Place a hand blender inside the jar. Mix the ingredients thoroughly. Season if necessary.

Heat your frying pan and melt the lard. Cook the pork chops for six minutes on each side. Boil a pot of water and blanch the asparagus for five minutes. Drain it afterwards.

Serve the pork chops with the asparagus spears. Put a drizzle of hollandaise over them.

3. Cheese and Tomato Omelet

Ingredients:

- 5 sprays of rapeseed oil
- 35 grams of cherry tomatoes (halved)
- ¼ red onion (finely diced)
- 6 fresh basil leaves
- 2 eggs
- 1 tablespoon of Parmesan cheese (grated)
- pepper
- salt

Instructions:

Heat a frying pan and spray rapeseed oil. Fry the red onion for five minutes. Add the cherry tomatoes. Cook for five more minutes. Remove the frying pan from the heat and add the basil leaves. Scoop out the tomato mixture and transfer it into a bowl.

In a separate bowl, place the eggs. Add some water. Mix them together. Add salt and pepper. Then, cook the beaten eggs on your frying pan. Add the Parmesan cheese and tomato mixture. Cook for another two minutes.

4. Fridge Salad

Ingredients:

- 40 grams of mixed salad leaves
- 1 carrot (grated)
- 2 spring onions (finely sliced)
- 3 baby plum tomatoes (halved)
- 8 slices of cucumber
- 38 grams of feta cheese
- 50 grams of pickled baby beets (halved)
- 1 tablespoon of balsamic vinegar
- black pepper

Instructions:

Put all ingredients on a plate. Top them with feta cheese and baby beets. Drizzle balsamic vinegar on top. Season with black pepper.

5. Tiger Prawn Curry with Basmati Rice

Ingredients:
- low fat cooking spray
- 1 teaspoon of black mustard seeds
- 2 chopped tomatoes
- 500 grams of raw tiger prawns (peeled)
- 100 grams of low fat yogurt
- 1 small coriander
- salt
- pepper

For the curry paste:
- 1 onion
- 4 cloves of garlic
- 2 red chillies
- 2 teaspoons of ground coriander
- 2 teaspoons of ground cumin
- 1 teaspoon of garam masala

- 1 teaspoon of chili powder
- ½ teaspoon of ground turmeric

For the curry sauce:
- salt
- lemon juice

Instructions:

Make a curry paste by mixing the ingredients in a food processor. Add one or two tablespoons of water. Mix all ingredients until they become smooth.

Heat a frying pan and spray it with the cooking spray. Fry the mustard seeds and add the curry sauce paste. Fry them for three more minutes. Add 250 ml. of water. Add the chopped tomatoes. Stir everything for five minutes.

Next, you should add the prawns. Simmer them for five minutes and then add salt and pepper to taste. Remove the frying pan from heat. Add the chopped coriander and yogurt.

6. Creamy Garlic Mushroom and Toast

Ingredients:

- 15 grams of margarine
- 1 clove of garlic
- 100 grams of mushrooms
- 20 grams of cream cheese
- 1 slice of wheat bread
- salt
- pepper

Instructions:

Heat a frying pan and melt the margarine. Cook the garlic for a minute before adding the mushrooms. Cook for five more minutes. Add the cream cheese. Cook for three more minutes. Season with salt and pepper.

Toast the wheat bread. Spread some margarine on it. Add the creamy garlic mushrooms.

7. Smoked Salmon Pita Pizza

Ingredients:
- 1 pita bread
- 1 tablespoon of low fat cream cheese
- 25 grams of smoked salmon
- ¼ red onion
- 1 teaspoon of drained capers
- 1 lemon wedge
- 40 grams of lettuce leaves
- 1 fresh dill

Instructions:

Preheat the oven to 180°C. Spread the low fat cream cheese on your pita bread and add some smoked salmon. Put a drizzle of chopped red onion on top of it. Add the drained capers. Bake everything for ten minutes. Check your pita bread every once in a while. Its edges should be crispy.

8. Herb and Spice Crusted Baked Chicken Breasts

Ingredients:

- Chicken breast fillets (boneless and skinless)
- 1 finely chopped oregano
- ¼ teaspoon of ground cumin
- ¼ teaspoon of ground coriander
- 250 grams of vegetable stock
- salt
- pepper
- chili powder
- low fat cooking spray

Instructions:

Preheat the oven to 200°C. Place the chicken breasts on a non-stick baking tray.

In a bowl, you have to mix the herbs and spices. Spread the mixture on the chicken breasts. Spray the low fat cooking spray on it. Pour the vegetable stock on your baking tray and bake the chicken breasts for twenty minutes.

They should be crispy and golden brown. Cut them into smaller pieces and serve with rice or vegetables.

9. Keto Cheeseburger

Ingredients:

For the burger patties:
- 1 tablespoon of lard
- 1 teaspoon of black pepper
- 1 teaspoon of salt
- 1 teaspoon of apple cider vinegar
- 1 clove of garlic
- 2 teaspoons of onion powder
- 600 grams of ground beef

For the burger sauce:
- 2 tablespoons of tomato puree
- ¼ cup of paleo mayonnaise
- 1 tablespoon of lemon juice

- pepper
- salt

For the burgers:
- 2 tablespoons of butter
- 4 nut-free keto buns
- 4 slices of bacon
- 16 slices of pickles
- 8 slices of red onion
- 4 slices of tomato
- 4 slices of cheddar cheese

Instructions:

Combine the ingredients for the burger patties in a bowl. Mix them well using your hands. You have to make four patties. Pierce them using a fork to loosen them up and allow them to cook evenly. Set aside.

In another bowl, you have to prepare the sauce. Mix the necessary ingredients and set them aside for a while.

Brown your keto burgers by cutting them widthwise and brushing them with melted butter. Cook them in a hot skillet for one minute. Remove them from the skillet and set them aside for a while.

Place some lard on your skillet. Cook the burger patties over high heat for three minutes. You should see crusts form at their bottoms. Cook them well, but refrain from piercing them with a fork. Cook the bacon slices on the same pan.

Assemble your burgers by spreading two teaspoons of burger sauce on the bun halves. Add slices of pickles and shredded lettuce. Add the burger patty, onions, tomatoes, and cheese slices. Place them in a broiler for one minute or until the cheese has melted. Top them with the cooked bacon.

Chapter 7: How to Gradually Transition to Intermittent Fasting

Switching to a new diet is not easy. Your body may undergo certain changes during the transition period. This is why you need to make sure that you prepare yourself well. Do not make sudden changes to avoid experiencing withdrawal symptoms. Make the change gradual.

Here are some tips on how you can do that:

Before you start intermittent fasting, you should consult your doctor. This is especially necessary if you have a pre-existing medical condition. If your doctor allows you to embark on this diet, you should keep things simple. Ideally, you should only drink water, unsweetened tea, or black coffee. You can eat your usual foods. Nonetheless, you may want to go for foods that are high in fat and low in carbohydrates.

Choose the time or schedule that works best for you. Likewise, you should choose the days that are most ideal. Many people prefer to fast on weekdays because these days have few variables and they are more structured. If you ever slip, do not beat yourself up. Remember that you are just a beginner. Forgive yourself for making a mistake and try again.

See to it that you also get clear with your purpose for embarking on intermittent fasting. Why are you on this diet? Are you trying to lose weight or maintain your current weight? Figure out what you want to achieve and focus on it. Intermittent fasting can help you lose weight and tone your body. It can also help you avoid diseases as well as lengthen your life span.

A Sample Week Plan

Now that you have an idea on how to get started, you can finally get down to it. You can use the following guide:

On your first day, you should not eat anything else after dinner time. This should not be a problem since you would be sleeping soon anyway. However, if you have to stay awake, make sure that you discipline yourself and not eat any midnight snacks. You can drink some tea or water to avoid getting hungry. You can also brush your teeth so that you can curb your cravings.

On your second day, you should delay breakfast. By this time, you have already had a twelve-hour fast. You can eat whenever it feels convenient for you, but it is more ideal to do it a couple of hours before lunch time. This way, you will not be tempted to have morning snacks. When you delay your breakfast, you can drink water, tea, or coffee. Then, you can have dinner. Do not eat anything else after that.

On your third day, you should not eat any snacks after lunch. Your next meal should be at dinner. To curb your cravings, you can drink water, tea, or coffee. You should also keep yourself busy to avoid thinking about food.

On your fourth day, you should skip breakfast. By this time, you have already had a fifteen-hour fast since you ate dinner last night. Your lunch or first meal of the day should be a little before noon or at about 11 AM. Then, you should have dinner and not eat any midnight snacks.

On your fifth day, you simply have to repeat the processes. You ate dinner last night and you skipped breakfast today. You ate lunch a little before noon and did not eat any snacks. You ate dinner at your usual schedule.

Chapter 8: How to Succeed – Effective Tips and Tricks and Hacks

You do not have to be a genius to succeed with intermittent fasting. You just have to have self-discipline, motivation, and focus. If you are truly determined to achieve your health goals, you will do everything you can.

Here are some tips, tricks, and hacks on how to make intermittent fasting work for you:

Focus on eating nutritious foods.

After you fasted for sixteen hours, you should not get complacent. Do not think that you can eat anything you want. You have to focus on your objectives. Remind yourself that you should only eat healthy foods.

Do not drink artificially flavored and sugary beverages.

While you are on intermittent fasting, you should only drink water, tea, or coffee. Refrain from drinking soda and energy drinks. Do not believe ads that claim certain beverages to be low in sugar. They have lots of artificial sweeteners. If the beverage is artificially flavored, it is not good for you. It can only make you hungrier and cause you to overeat.

Drink sufficient amounts of water.

Make sure that you keep your body hydrated by drinking enough water. You can also suppress your appetite by drinking water before you eat. If you find plain water boring, you can add some fruit slices to give it flavor.

Stay busy while fasting.

If you do not have anything worthwhile to do, you will just keep thinking about food. This is why you need to keep yourself busy. Focus on your work or start a new hobby. Do something that can distract you from thinking about food.

Exercise

Of course, you also need to exercise. Diet and exercise go hand in hand. If you want to achieve your fitness goals, you need to exercise on a regular basis. Ideally, you should combine cardio and strength training exercises.

Get sufficient rest and sleep.

Do not overwork yourself. Make sure that you rest and sleep. Remember that your body burns calories while it performs certain functions during sleep. You need to sleep in order to improve your metabolism and reduce your risk of diseases.

Conclusion

Now that you have reached the Conclusion part, I would like to congratulate and thank you for downloading this book.

I hope that it was able to boost your knowledge about dieting and living a healthy lifestyle. More importantly, I hope that it was able to provide you with all the information you need about intermittent fasting.

Intermittent fasting is indeed an effective method for losing weight and improving your health. It is simple, straightforward, and easy. It does not involve any complex routines. You simply have to watch what you eat and be mindful of when to eat.

Then again, it is still important to consult your doctor before you go through this diet. Make sure that you also transition from your old diet to this new diet properly to avoid experiencing withdrawal symptoms. With discipline and determination, you can surely achieve your desired results using intermittent fasting.

The next step is to apply the lessons that you have learned from this book into your life. Do not forget to share your newfound knowledge with your family and friends. Encourage them to get this book as well.

Thank you and good luck!

Part 2

The 5:2 Diet simply defined:

This diet is sometimes known as the Fasting Diet, the Intermittent Fasting Diet or the Fasting and Feasting Diet. They all come down to the same principle, though I prefer to drop the word "fasting" as it can convey a misleading (and perhaps off-putting) impression.

☐ *You choose **any** two days per week you wish and cut the total number of calories consumed on those days to a quarter of the recommended daily amount. So if you are female you can eat 500 and if you are male it's 600 calories for each of those days. You can change those days around as you wish each week to fit in with your social calendar. The only rule to this is that the days are not consecutive.*

☐ *It is completely up to you whether to skip breakfast and/or lunch, reserving all or most of your calories for your evening meal; or to consume the bulk of your day's calories for breakfast. Alternatively, you can spread your calories to allow for three meals on your low-calorie days. This book is designed for this last option, though you can, if you wish, simply select one or two recipes from any day and supplement your intake with drinks or your own recipe to add up to your daily allowance. Just click on the title of any recipe in the index to take you directly to it. You have total control over the way you do the 5:2 diet.*

☐ No food as such is banned from your two low calorie days so long as it doesn't exceed the target number of calories.

☐ On the other five days of your week you can please yourself what you eat or drink. Chocolate, wine, cakes... all these treats are permitted, although it makes good sense to consume them in moderation. I know of no other diet that is as flexible about food.

☐On the 5:2 diet no food is classed as a "sin", allowed only in small amounts or completely forbidden.

*

Impressive ways in which this novel way of eating could change your life forever:

☐Your weight loss is guaranteed if you stick to the principles outlined within these pages. This benefit will undoubtedly be the first to become apparent. You can be confident that you are on the path to banishing those unwanted pounds of fat forever! In itself this is sufficiently rewarding to encourage you to carry on even before you reap the other benefits.

☐You will ultimately feel more energised.

☐Exercising will become easier as you will have less weight to carry around.

☐ *Your appetite on the five "normal" days of eating will gradually decrease as your stomach shrinks and you feel less need for large amounts of food.*

☐ *It will quite possibly prevent the mental deterioration that we are all prone to develop with age – Alzheimer's disease, dementia, Parkinson's disease... An enormous amount of research has been done over several years, with rodents, to back up this claim. And, even if you are not a rodent results are promising; the increasing numbers of human studies substantiate the findings with animals.*

☐ *Just two days each week involving lowered calorie intake can make all the difference to how healthily we live our lives. It could also dramatically increase our longevity. This is because the level of a growth hormone called the IGF1 hormone, which tends to be produced in large amounts as we age, is automatically lowered when we calorie restrict. This reduction triggers the body into repairing existing damaged cells rather than focus on new cell manufacture. Once this occurs, harm that may have been done to your body over the years can, in this marvellous work of reparation, actually begin to reverse the damage done to your body in the past, giving you renewed hope for a healthier and hopefully, happier future!*

☐ Hunger appears to make the brain more alert, though in the early weeks of the diet you will probably experience short-lived hunger pangs until your body adjusts. These can easily be soothed with plenty of calorie- free cold drinks of health-giving water and/or hot, non-calorie drinks such as black or green tea. So your memory power should improve and your ability to think sharpen considerably.

☐ Eating the 5:2 way can normalise blood sugar, avoiding the danger of type 2 diabetes, which is usually associated with obesity in adulthood.

☐ *Cholesterol levels can be lowered, thereby significantly diminishing the risks of developing heart disease.*

☐ *Research strongly suggests that keeping to the 5:2 diet plan can play an important role in preventing development of various cancers and other serious diseases. Once again, human research in this area, though not yet extensive, supports the outcomes of animal studies.*

We could well be on the brink of an exciting breakthrough in this aspect of research. Already we are aware of a group of approximately three hundred people in the world who have what is termed 'Laron's Syndrome'. These individuals are born without the growth-related IGF1 hormone and grow to less than four feet as adults. So, not having the hormone is a disadvantage when they are young. However, despite their shortness of height they all live long, reasonably healthy lives without suffering from the diseases we usually associate with aging. Indeed, were it not for the fact the some of them drink alcohol excessively and smoke, who knows how much longer they might live?

To summarise: by following the 5:2 diet it would seem that we stand a far better than average chance of living longer, active, disease-free lives. Who could realistically ask for more, except perhaps to win the lottery...

Now you are equipped with all the important basic facts you need to know to begin the 5:2 diet.

To help you on your way, this book contains twenty each of recipes for vegetarian breakfasts, lunches and suppers, complete with calorie counts at the start of each meal and the total for each day. A man's extra 100 calorie allowance can easily be topped up, using these recipes, with an added portion of vegetables (vegetables being on the whole low calorie means he could have a reasonably generous portion) or a low calorie snack. A few of the meals I have included can simply be doubled in quantity.

Important Note

It is essential to mention at this point that there are a few groups of people for whom this diet is definitely unsuitable. They are:

- *Pregnant or breastfeeding women*
- *Children*
- *Diabetics*
- *Anyone with a history of eating disorders*

However, anyone who has a health condition for which they are being treated by their GP should discuss the wisdom, or not, of proceeding with this or any other diet.

My Personal Experience

The 5:2 diet is not a really hard diet to stick to. Eight months on, I can state this with absolute assurance and conviction. Yet, before beginning the 5:2 diet, I had never stayed on **any** diet for more than a few weeks, at the very most. Every one I came across involved a strong dose of sustained willpower. It had taken me many years to quit smoking and I was not prepared to undertake anything that was equally difficult. So, after searching for several years for **the** diet that could suit my love of food and lack of commitment, I was fast reaching the conclusion that there was, in fact, no such diet – until the 5:2 hit the scene.

Although I already possessed a blender I treated myself to a juicer and citrus squeezer to make life that much easier. And I mustered up every bit of enthusiasm I could, determined to apply myself single-mindedly to my first day of calorie restricting. After a weekend of my usual comfort eating, I began.

When I first started, though, I was more than a little concerned that 500 calories would consist of far too little to fill me up for a day. I was slightly horrified when I found out that the baked potato with cheese and baked beans I was planning for my evening meal on the first day totalled a massive 532 calories – more than my allotted allowance for the entire day! Additionally, when I totted up the number of calories I had already consumed by suppertime, it came to 320, even though I thought I had been pretty meagre in my choice – a glass of orange juice and a slice of wholemeal bread spread with peanut butter for breakfast and only a pear for lunch.

Perhaps this diet, that so many people I knew were enthusing about, was not for me. Maybe, I would just have to resign myself to being five stone overweight, I thought unhappily. But my husband's promise of a summer holiday in the South of France the following year, to celebrate our fifteenth wedding anniversary, spurred me on. I wanted so much to fit comfortably into that seat on the plane and not attract stares as I ventured onto the beach in my swimming costume.

I decided that I would keep going with this diet for a month and if, by then, I was finding it unbearably hard I would abandon it and wait for the next new diet to come along.

I began to plan my two low calorie days carefully in advance, working out the calorie content of each recipe I used. The problem was that, although my husband is also a vegetarian, he had no intention of doing this diet with me. To be honest, he's not overweight and he said he wasn't going to start dieting in the hope of living a few years longer; he also told me that I looked beautiful, whatever my size.

Despite his compliment, I sat down and added my doctor's recent stern warning - that I was on track to develop diabetes if I did not cut down on the amount I ate - to my list of incentives to get started. I would go it alone.

During the first few weeks I have to admit that I hit a number of obstacles, quite apart from what food to put on my plate on a calorie restricted day.

Initially, I was missing meals, usually breakfast, and feeling totally lacking in energy. So I began to work on having three daily as I had been used to. This is, after all, not meant to be a starvation diet and eating my usual number of meals made the whole experience feel more familiar to me.

As my low calorie day wore on I found I began to get a headache. When I mentioned this to one of my friends who started the diet around the same time I did, she suggested drinking a glass of water before each meal and a few more glasses than I normally did during the day; this seemed to do the trick and the energy dips stopped also .

Another problem was that, although I knew it was a good idea to increase my fluid intake, I wasn't sure, at first, what I could drink throughout the day, other than water, without adding to the calories. So I did a bit of research and compiled a list of calorie-free drinks to choose from, (you'll find it at the beginning of the next section).

If I got to the end of one of my two days feeling tired and/or a bit unsure whether I had the stamina to continue with this diet, I would have an early night and console myself with the thought that the next day I could eat whatever I wished.

Oddly enough though, I found after the first couple of weeks that I no longer had the voracious craving for food I've had for years. I would prepare a meal, on my 'normal' days, only to find I couldn't eat more than half of it. This reduction in appetite was an unexpected but welcome bonus, though it's quite logical if I'd stopped to think about it.

<u>As the weeks turned into months I encountered a further effect of my altered style of eating: my</u> size 20 clothes were ill fitting and unflattering. Time I would once have spent snacking on calorie laden snacks got used up browsing clothes shops for some new, more attractive items of clothing. Busying myself on my low calorie days was, for me, an important way to cope whilst following my new eating patterns. I enjoy cooking and focused far more on shopping for ingredients and making my meals than I had done previously. Sometimes, when a hunger pang struck (and they did quite often in those early weeks) I would <u>distract myself with my watercolours, immerse myself in a good book or concentrate on writing. And,</u>

<u>any time I saw someone eating a cream cake or an ice cream, I would remind myself that I only had to wait until my twenty-four hours were up to indulge if I felt so inclined. That way I did not feel I was missing out.</u>

Instead of adding calorie–laden sugar to a recipe I sometimes substituted stevia, a totally natural plant extract with zero calories (a third of a teaspoon is equivalent to a full teaspoon of granulated sugar). Surprisingly, however, my cravings for sweet foods have decreased dramatically.

A further couple of notes on substitution – I find that liquid egg white can sometimes be an excellent alternative to eggs; besides being only 15 calories instead of 55 where a small egg might be used, it is much lower in cholesterol.

And I found that having a one calorie oil spray in stock is especially useful, particularly when you realise that a tablespoon of olive oil is 120 calories.

My weight loss has been slow but steady and I find it a lot easier to move around and so do more exercise than before I started this diet. I actually feel energetic, a word I never dreamed I would ever use with reference to myself. I look forward to my low calorie days and they never interfere with my social life – any time I go out to eat I simply swap the days around, if necessary, for that week. In fact, I rarely keep to the same two days, preferring to remain completely flexible about my weekly scheduling. And I have noticed an improvement in my mood, perhaps, in no small part, because I am now within healthy weight limits and physically lighter.

I am still enjoying the 5:2 diet, still finding it rewarding (not least the prospect of this slimmer, more energetic me walking along the beach in Cannes in August) and have every intention of continuing indefinitely. It's a lifestyle choice that I am glad I made. I was amazed, after only eight months, when I jumped on the scales for my weekly weigh-in, to discover that I had achieved my goal – I was five stone lighter than when I began the diet! It was a great moment. If you had asked me a year ago if I thought it was possible I would have laughed or groaned, or both. I immediately rang two of my friends, who are also on the 5:2 diet, with the good news. The three of us have cajoled, encouraged and praised each other along the way.

So finally, here it is the diet that suits me and I'm sure will suit you.

My journey, so far, has inspired me to write this book. If I can do this diet, you can too!

Calorie-Free Drinks (or almost!)

The following is a list of drinks that are either completely calorie free or no more than a couple of calories each. This list is obviously not exhaustive, but will at least provide you with a few ideas for drinks for your 2 calorie restricted days.

Water (tap or bottled)

Sparkling water

Diet cola

Diet soda

Iced tea

Black tea

Green tea

Earl Grey tea

Rooibos tea (Red Bush)

Vast variety of fruit teas / fruit infusions (1-3 calories)

You can make your own flavoured water by taking a large jug of cold water and adding slices of low calorie fruit or vegetables, such as cucumber, lemons or strawberries, or herbs, such as mint or basil. These are virtually calorie-free drinks.

Breakfast

Poached Eggs with Mushrooms: 135 calories

1 slice wholemeal bread

1 small egg
1 drop of vinegar

Pinch of salt

56g (2 oz) button mushrooms, wiped clean with a damp paper towel

1- cal vegetable oil spray

Bring to the boil a half-filled medium saucepan of salted water.

Put a slice of toast into a toaster

Spray a frying pan with 4 sprays of 1-cal oil and heat gently

Break the egg into a cup and add a drop of vinegar (this helps the egg to keep its shape in the pan).

Whisk or stir the boiling water vigorously to make it swirl and drop the egg into the middle.

Reduce the heat to low and cook for about three minutes.

Meanwhile, fry the mushrooms on a medium heat, keeping them moving in the pan until golden (approximately 3 minutes).

Use a slotted spoon to remove the egg from the water and drain on a piece of kitchen towel

Place the egg in the centre of the toast, surround with the mushrooms and serve immediately.

Lunch

Quick Bruschetta: 204 calories

84g (3 oz) tomatoes, chopped

14g (½ oz) red onion, finely chopped

½ small clove of garlic, crushed

1 tsp olive oil

Tiny sprinkle sugar – edge of tsp

3 large leaves fresh basil, chopped

1 thick slice of crusty bread

10ml (2 tsp) olive oil for the bread

Mix together all the ingredients except the bread and 10ml olive oil.

Drizzle 10ml olive oil on the bread.

Lightly toast bread on both sides under the grill.

Spread mixture evenly on toasted bread and serve.

Use knife and fork to eat.

Supper

Cauliflower Bake: 157 calories

1 small potato, cubed
3 oz (84g) cauliflower florets
3 cherry tomatoes

Sauce:
1 tsp butter
1 baby leek, chopped
½ small clove garlic, chopped
1 level tsp plain flour
60ml (2 fl.oz) almond milk
14g (½ oz) grated Parmesan-style vegetarian cheese
Small pinch paprika

Preheat oven to 350°F/175 °C/Gas Mark 5
Boil potato cubes in pan of water until cooked but firm.
Steam cauliflower until tender (about 4 minutes).

Sauce:

Melt butter in a pan, add leek and garlic and sauté for 1 minute.

Stir in the flour until smoothly blended.

Remove the pan from heat and slowly add the almond milk, stirring continuously.

Add cheese and paprika.

Put the cauliflower in small ovenproof dish with cherry tomatoes and cooked potatoes.

Stir in the sauce

Bake for about 12 minutes until thoroughly heated.

Day 2: 495 calories

Breakfast

Apple and walnut Porridge: 159 calories

10g (1/3 oz) porridge oats
10g (1/3 oz) raisins

10g (1/3 oz) chopped walnuts

60ml (2 fl.oz) pure apple juice

Mix all ingredients well in a microwaveable bowl.

Microwave for 1½ minutes (based on 700W – adjust time accordingly).

Stir and serve.

Lunch

Asparagus Omelette: 100 calories

1-cal olive oil spray

1 large egg

1 tsp finely chopped herbs, fresh

Salt and ground black pepper

5 asparagus tips

3 cherry tomatoes, halved

Sprig of parsley

Cook asparagus in a few inches of boiling water in a covered saucepan for about 8 minutes until the tips are tender.

Drain, return to pan and cover to keep warm.

Coat an omelette pan with 4 sprays of 1-cal olive oil and heat gently over medium heat.

Whisk egg.

Add herbs, salt and pepper to taste.

Pour mixture into pan and spread evenly.

When set, and golden on the underside, arrange asparagus on one side and fold omelette in half.

Slide onto warmed plate, garnish with parsley and decorate with tomatoes.

Supper

Stir Fry Bok Choy: 236 calories

112g (4 oz) firm tofu, drained
½ tbsp hulled sesame seeds

2 tsp toasted sesame oil, divided

170g (6 oz) large bok choy, chopped

28g (1 oz) cooked black beans

1 small clove garlic, minced

½ tbsp minced fresh ginger

½ tsp dark brown sugar

½ tbsp low-sodium tamari

A few drops of chilli-garlic sauce

Cut tofu into small cubes.

Roll cubes in sesame seeds.

Heat 1 tsp sesame oil in a non-stick frying pan over a medium heat.

Add tofu, and cook until golden brown (approx. 10 min.), turning occasionally. Put to one side.

Heat remaining oil in a wok over high heat.

Stir-fry the bok choy for 4 minutes.

Add black beans, garlic and ginger and continue to stir-fry for a further 2 minutes.

Stir in brown sugar and tamari, then add chilli-garlic sauce

Fold in the tofu before serving.

Day 3: 495 calories

Breakfast

Apple and Cucumber Refresher: 60 calories

70ml (2½ fl.oz) pure apple juice
112g (4 oz) cucumber, peeled and chopped
5g fresh mint, chopped
5 ice cubes

Pour the apple juice into a blender.
Add the cucumber and mint and ice cubes.
Blend on a high setting until completely smooth.
Pour into a glass and serve immediately.

This is a refreshing start to a summer morning!

Lunch

Sweet and Savoury Salad: 240 calories

1 small orange, segmented
56 g (2 oz) strawberries, halved
56 g (2 oz) mixed salad leaves
10 g toasted pecan nuts

Cinnamon & Ginger Vinaigrette:

2 tsp olive oil
2 tsp orange juice
¼ tsp ground ginger
¼ tsp ground cinnamon
Stevia to taste
Sea salt and black pepper to taste

Combine the salad ingredients in a bowl.

Make the vinaigrette, by mixing all its ingredients together well.

Pour the vinaigrette over the salad and toss the salad to ensure even coating.

Serve immediately.

Supper

Cheese & Onion Frittata: 195 calories

3 tablespoons "2 Chicks" liquid egg white*

30ml (2 tbsp) semi-skimmed milk

5ml (1 tsp) fresh parsley, chopped

Salt and freshly ground pepper to taste

1 small carrot, chopped

½ small onion, chopped

28g (1 oz) cheddar cheese, grated

1-cal olive oil spray

This quantity is based on "2 Chicks" Liquid Egg White and is equivalent to 1 egg. Other brands may vary.

Whisk together the egg white, milk, parsley, salt and pepper.

Coat a small omelette pan with 6 sprays of 1-cal olive oil spray and heat gently.

Fry the carrot and onion for a few minutes until tender.

Pour egg mixture over vegetables and sprinkle with cheese.

Cook on a low heat for approx. 5 minutes until the mixture has set and the underside is golden brown.

Transfer to a warmed plate for serving.

Day 4: 500 calories

Breakfast

Fruity Oatbars: 135 calories in 1 bar
(Makes 8, 1 to eat now, the rest to wrap and freeze)

84g (3 oz) rolled oats

½ tsp almond extract

2 tbsp honey

56g (2 oz) peanut butter

56g (2 oz) chopped almonds

28g (1 oz) flax seeds

1 tsp cinnamon

¼ tsp nutmeg

1 tsp vanilla extract

½ small banana

Combine all ingredients until well mixed.

Spread the mixture evenly into a small baking tin and press down well.

Place in freezer for approximately 1 hour, until firm.

Slice into 8 equal bars.

Foil-wrap all but one and freeze until required.

Lunch

Fresh Fruit Salad: 175 calories

28g (1 oz) blueberries
1 medium plum, stoned and chopped
1 satsuma, segmented
1 apricot, halved
1 small banana, sliced
84g (3 oz) strawberries, sliced
5 seedless grapes
Small wedge honeydew melon, cubed
Juice of 1 lemon, freshly squeezed
Stevia to taste

Combine all the fruit in a bowl.
Pour lemon juice over and mix well.
Sweeten with stevia as required.
Serve at room temperature or chill if preferred.

Supper

Scrambled Egg with Chives: 190 calories

2 small eggs
15ml (½ fl oz) skimmed milk
2g (½ tsp) butter
1 slice wholemeal bread
¼ tsp oregano
2 fresh chives, finely chopped
Sea salt and white pepper to season

Whisk eggs and milk vigorously.
Season with salt and pepper.
Toast bread on both sides.
Melt butter gently in saucepan over low heat.
Add egg mixture and increase heat to medium.
Stir until cooked to desired consistency.

Sprinkle with oregano and remove from heat.

Top the toast evenly with the egg.

Garnish with chives.

Day 5: 500 Calories

Breakfast

Hot Grain Breakfast: 188 calories

60ml (2 fl.oz) fat free milk

28g (1 oz) couscous

28g (2 oz) raisins

28g (1 oz) blueberries

Stevia to taste

Microwave milk until hot (about 40 seconds or less, depending on your microwave).

Add couscous to milk and allow to stand for 5 minutes.

Stir in raisins and blueberries.

Add stevia to taste.

Lunch

Fruit & Ginger Smoothie: 128 calories

1 passion fruit

56g (2 oz) prepacked fresh or frozen mango slices

1 extra small banana

60ml (2 fl.oz) apple juice

½ tsp ground ginger

Ice cubes (optional)

Cut passion fruit in half, scoop out the flesh and seeds and discard the shell.

Place all ingredients into a blender.

Blend thoroughly until smooth.

Add ice if desired and serve

Supper

Spinach & Onion Omelette: 184 calories

1-cal olive oil

2 tbsp chopped onion

½ tsp dried Italian seasoning

28 g (1 oz) torn spinach leaves

2 medium eggs

Pinch ground black pepper

2 tbsp (½ oz.) shredded part-skimmed mozzarella cheese

-

Coat an omelette pan with 6 sprays of olive oil over medium heat.

Add onion and Italian seasoning and fry until onion is tender (approx. 3 min).

Add spinach leaves and cook briefly until they wilt (approx. 1 min).

Remove from heat and set mixture on a plate to one side.

Respray pan with 4 sprays of olive oil and place over medium heat.

Whisk the eggs and add pepper.

Pour the egg mixture into the pan and cook until it begins to set and the underside is golden brown.

Place the vegetable mixture and cheese on one half of the egg and fold the other half over.

Allow to cook for a further minute to allow the cheese to melt.

Slide onto a plate and serve while hot.

Day 6: 497 calories

Breakfast

Oatmeal & Blueberry Breakfast: 95 calories

10g (1/3 oz) porridge oats
Pinch of cinnamon
56g (2 oz) blueberries

60ml soya milk

Mix oats with cinnamon and soya milk.
Microwave for 1½ minutes (based on 700W – adjust accordingly).
Add blueberries and stir.
Microwave for 30 seconds.
Stir and serve.

Lunch

Miso Aubergines: 153 calories

1 small aubergine, halved lengthways
1-cal olive oil
Sea salt
Ground pepper
1 tbsp miso paste
1 tbsp apple juice
Pinch of stevia

½ tbsp lemon juice

½ tbsp sesame seeds

2 spring onions, chopped

Rocket (arugula) leaves, small handful

Preheat oven to 200ºC/390ºF/Gas Mark 6.

Use a sharp knife to score the flesh of the aubergine halves with a criss-cross pattern.

Spray each half with 3 sprays of oil and season with salt and pepper.

Place on non stick baking tray and roast for 20 minutes.

Heat grill to high temperature.

Mix miso and apple juice with stevia and lemon juice.

Spread the mixture over cooked aubergines.

Sprinkle with sesame seeds.

Grill until golden, 2-3 minutes.

Serve on a bed of rocket leaves and garnished with spring onions.

Supper

Lemon and Parsley Couscous: 249 calories

60g (2 oz) couscous
210ml (7 fl.oz) vegetable stock, boiling
1 small tomato, chopped
28g (1 oz) pomegranate seeds
28g (1 oz) spring onions, finely sliced
Pinch garlic granules
Pinch dried chillies, crushed
½ tsp parsley, chopped
2 tsp lemon juice
2 tsp olive oil
28g (1 oz) light halloumi cheese
Sea salt
Black pepper

Place couscous in a pan or heatproof bowl and pour in the vegetable stock.

Add the remaining ingredients except lemon juice, olive oil and halloumi, salt and pepper.

Cover and put to one side for 10 minutes.

Slice halloumi.

Heat oil in non-stick frying pan and fry halloumi slices until golden on both sides.

Fluff couscous with a fork.

Drizzle couscous with lemon juice, add salt and pepper and toss lightly.

Serve with halloumi slices.

Day 7: 499 calories

Breakfast

Carrot and Mango Crush: 185 calories

28g (2 oz) prepacked fresh mango slices

75ml (2½ fl.oz) freshly-squeezed orange juice

30ml (1 fl.oz) carrot juice

Crushed ice, to serve

Rocket (arugula) leaves, to decorate

Place all ingredients, except ice and rocket, into a blender.

Blend until smooth.

Pour into tall glass, stir in ice and top with rocket leaves.

Lunch

Spicy Onion & Tomato Salad: 47 calories

1 very small onion, sliced

1 medium vine tomato, sliced

¼ green chilli, deseeded and finely chopped

½ tbsp lemon juice

¼ tsp coriander leaf, finely chopped

Sea salt to taste

Mix together tomato and onion slices and chopped chilli.

Stir in lemon juice, coriander leaf and salt.

Refrigerate for approximately an hour and serve chilled.

Supper

Feta Tortilla Wrap: 267 calories

1 10-inch whole-wheat tortilla

42 g (1½ oz) feta cheese, crumbled

2 black olives, sliced

¼ small yellow squash, sliced

¼ cucumber, diced

4 cherry tomatoes, halved

1 very small red onion, thinly sliced

2 tsp balsamic vinegar

½ small clove garlic, minced

2 tsp chopped fresh parsley

½ tsp olive oil

Sea salt

Black ground pepper

Mix all ingredients apart from tortilla in a bowl.

Allow to stand for 15 minutes, stirring occasionally.

Drain off liquid and place mixture on tortilla.

Fold bottom of wrap over lower part of filling.

Roll up the tortilla to form a wrap.

-

Day 8: 499 Calories

Breakfast

Spiced Fruit Smoothie: 192 calories

½ small banana, sliced
½ ripe pear, peeled and diced
1 small apple, peeled and diced
75ml (2½ fl.oz) apple juice
75ml (2½ fl.oz) low-fat vanilla yoghurt
Pinch of ground cinnamon

Mint leaves

Ice cubes

Place all ingredients, except mint and ice cubes, into a blender.

Whizz until smooth.

Pour into tall glass.

Add ice and top with mint leaves.

Lunch

Tomatoes with Okra & Onion: 71 calories

1-cal olive oil spray

1 small onion, chopped

½ clove garlic, crushed

Pinch cayenne pepper (go easy!)

½ green pepper, chopped

70g (2½ oz) okra, sliced

56g (2 oz) canned, chopped tomatoes with juice

1 fresh tomato, chopped

Sea salt

Ground black pepper

Coat frying pan with 6 sprays olive oil and heat over medium heat.

Add onion, garlic, green pepper, okra and cayenne pepper and cook until tender (approx. 4 minutes), stirring continuously.

Add canned tomatoes and juice and fresh tomato, season with salt and pepper.

Reduce heat to low and simmer until all vegetables are tender (approx. 4 minutes).

Supper

Vegetable Broth: 236 calories

2 tsp vegetable oil

1 small onion, chopped

1 tsp chopped rosemary

½ small garlic clove, chopped

1 small carrot, chopped

215ml vegetable stock

100g can chickpeas, drained

25g green beans, chopped

Heat the oil in a small pan over a medium heat.

Add onion, rosemary and garlic and fry for 2 minutes.

Add carrots and pour in stock.

Simmer for 10 minutes before mixing in the chickpeas.

Stir in the beans and simmer for a further 3 minutes.

Day 9: 500 calories

Breakfast

Blueberry-Packed Smoothie: 160 calories

120 ml (4 fl.oz) fat-free natural yoghurt

75 ml (2½ fl.oz) pure apple juice
150 g (5 oz) fresh blueberries
Stevia to sweeten according to taste
Ice as desired

Put yoghurt, apple juice and blueberries into a blender.
Blend until smooth.
Add stevia to taste and blend again briefly.
Add ice and pour into a tall glass.

Lunch

Edamame Salad: 127 calories

56 g (2 oz) shelled edamame, fresh or frozen
28 g (1 oz) thinly sliced red cabbage
½ small orange pepper, thinly sliced
40g (1½ oz) finely diced pineapple
10g golden raisins
3g almonds, chopped

1 tsp fresh mint, chopped

1 tsp fresh lime juice

1 tsp honey

2 drops chile-garlic sauce

Boil edamame beans for 5 minutes (10 min. if frozen).

Drain and rinse with cold water.

Place edamame in a bowl and add the remaining ingredients.

Mix well before serving.

Supper

Chinese Ginger Vegetables: 213 calories

1-cal olive oil spray

½ inch fresh ginger, peeled & grated

1 small onion, sliced thinly

150g (5 oz) frozen mixed vegetables

56g (2 oz) fresh or frozen French beans, sliced

75ml (2½ fl.oz) water

1 tbsp dark brown sugar

1 tbsp cornflour

2 tbsp soy sauce

2 tbsp malt vinegar

½ tsp ground ginger

Coat large frying pan with 6 sprays of oil over medium heat.

Add ginger, fry for 1 minute.

Remove from pan and drain on piece of kitchen towelling and place to one side.

Place vegetables and water in the frying pan.

Cover, and cook for 5 – 6 minutes until vegetables are tender.

In a bowl, combine sugar, cornflour, soy sauce, malt vinegar and ground ginger.

Add this mix to the vegetables in the frying pan and simmer, whilst stirring, for 1 minute until liquid thickens.

Stir in the grated ginger.

Cook for a further two minutes before serving.

Day 10: 499 calories

Breakfast

Blueberry Quark Pancake: 130 calories

40g ((1½ oz) quark
3 tablespoons liquid egg-white*
100ml (3½ fl.oz) water
1 pinch salt
<u>20g (¾ oz) plain flour</u>
28g (1 oz) blueberries
Stevia to taste
1-cal olive oil spray

This quantity is based on "2 Chicks" Liquid Egg White and is equivalent to 1 egg. Other brands may vary.

Whisk together quark, egg white, water, salt and flour.

Allow batter to stand for 10 minutes.

Coat small non-stick omelette pan with 4 sprays of 1-cal oil and heat on high temperature.

Reduce heat to medium and pour in batter to cover pan evenly.

Cook for approximately 3 minutes until almost set

Loosen edges with spatula and cook until the base is golden brown (1 – 2 minutes)

Sprinkle blueberries onto one half.

Add stevia to taste.

Fold carefully in half and slide onto warmed plate.

Lunch

Fresh Mediterranean Salad: 132 calories

6 Romaine lettuce leaves, torn

10 slices cucumber

½ small green pepper, sliced

2 cherry tomatoes, halved

½ very small onion, sliced into rings

2 radishes, thinly sliced

1 tsp fresh parsley, chopped

½ pita bread

Dressing:

7½ ml (1½ tsp) lemon juice
7½ ml (1½ tsp) olive oil
tiny piece garlic clove, crushed
2 mint leaves, finely chopped
sea salt
black pepper

Put all salad ingredients in a bowl and mix gently.

Thoroughly mix lemon juice, olive oil, garlic, mint, salt and pepper.

Pour dressing over salad and lightly toss to coat.

Serve with warmed pita bread.

Supper

Carrot & Lentil Soup: 237 calories

½ tsp cumin seeds

Very small pinch chilli flakes

½ tbsp olive oil

150g (5½ oz) grated carrot

35g (1½ oz) split red lentils

35 ml (1½ fl.oz) semi-skimmed or soya milk

250ml (8½ fl.oz) vegetable stock

1 tsp plain fat free yoghurt

5 coriander leaves, torn

Dry-fry cumin seeds and chilli flakes in a hot saucepan for approx 1 minute until you can smell the aroma.

Add oil, carrot, lentils, milk and vegetable stock and bring to the boil.

Reduce heat and simmer for 15 minutes until lentils are softened.

Serve, topped with yoghurt and coriander leaves.

Day 11: 500 calories

Breakfast

Orange Fruit Salad: 120 calories

1 large orange, peeled and cut horizontally into slices

40 ml (1½ fl.oz) orange juice

½ tsp mint, chopped

¼ tsp ground cinnamon

mint leaves to garnish

Mix together orange slices, orange juice and chopped mint in serving bowl.

Sprinkle with cinnamon.

Garnish with mint leaves.

Lunch

Red Pepper Soup: 77 calories

180ml (6 fl.oz) vegetable stock
½ red pepper
½ small onion
1 tiny clove garlic
1 small tomato, halved

Preheat oven to 180°C/350°F/Gas mark 4.

Place pepper, onion, garlic and tomato on a foil lined baking tray.

Roast for 10 minutes.

Remove skin from tomato and squeeze garlic from its skin.

Put all ingredients including stock in a blender and blend until smooth.

Pour into saucepan, heat gently and serve.

   Supper

Stuffed Pepper: 303 calories

1 medium red pepper, cut in half, lengthways and deseeded

56g (2 oz) couscous

1-calorie olive oil spray

1 very small onion, chopped

Juice and zest of ½ lemon

28g (1 oz) reduced fat feta cheese, crumbled

½ tsp ground coriander

1 dried apricot, chopped

Preheat oven to 200°C, 400°F, Gas Mark 6.

Place pepper halves on a baking tray (oiled or non-stick) and cook for 10 minutes until tender.

Meanwhile, pour 60 ml boiling water over the couscous, cover and leave for 10 minutes until absorbed.

Coat a small frying pan with 6 sprays of 1-calorie olive oil and heat gently.

Fry the onion, stirring constantly, for approx. 3 minutes until softened.

Add lemon juice and zest, feta cheese, coriander, apricot and onion to the couscous.

Stuff the roasted peppers with the couscous mixture and serve.

Day 12: 492 calories

Breakfast

Spiced Fruit Salad: 70 calories

56g (2 oz) melon
56g (2 oz) strawberries
56g (2 oz) grapes
56g (2 oz) apple slices
56g (2 oz) blackberries
¼ tsp mixed spice

Cut the melon into small chunks.
Slice the strawberries.
Halve the grapes.
Mix all fruit in a bowl with mixed spice.

Serve at room temperature or chilled.

Lunch

Summer Salad: 83 calories

70g cumber, peeled
2 medium tomatoes
20 g orange pepper
3 basil leaves
¼ clove garlic
1 tsp cider vinegar
½ tsp olive oil
sea salt
black pepper

Chop cucumber, tomatoes, pepper and basil into small pieces.
Mix with remainder of the ingredients and chill in refrigerator for 30 minutes.
Serve cold.

Supper

Twirly Pasta with Tomatoes, Spinach & Cheese: 339 calories

56g (2 oz) pasta twirls, cooked and drained
¾ tbsp olive oil
¾ tbsp white wine vinegar
¼ tsp thyme
¼ tsp rosemary
pinch garlic granules
pinch basil
pinch oregano
Sea salt to taste
14g (½ oz) baby spinach leaves
28g (1 oz) light mozzarella cheese, torn
½ tsp Parmesan-style vegetarian cheese, grated
56g (2 oz) cherry tomatoes, halved

Mix together oil, vinegar, thyme, rosemary, garlic, basil, oregano and sea salt.

Add cooked pasta and spinach and toss thoroughly.

Mix in cheeses and tomatoes.

Serve warm or allow to cool according to preference.

Day 13: 500 calories

Breakfast

Peanut Butter and Fruit Waffle: 165 calories

1 low fat waffle

½ tbsp peanut butter

½ small banana, sliced

2 strawberries, sliced

Toast the waffle on both sides.

Spread the peanut butter evenly on the waffle.

Decorate with alternate slices of banana and strawberries.

Lunch

Spicy Cauliflower: 140 calories

1-cal olive oil spray

¼ tsp cumin seeds

¼ small green chilli, chopped

¼ tsp chopped fresh ginger

½ tsp garlic pulp

120g (4 oz) cauliflower florets

Pinch ground turmeric

28g (1 oz) peas

Small pinch garam masala

Small pinch ground cumin

½ tbsp fresh coriander, chopped

1 tsp lemon juice

Heat 10 sprays olive oil in a wok over a medium heat.

Put in cumin seeds, chilli, ginger and garlic and stir well.

Add cauliflower, turmeric and peas.

Sprinkle with a little water and cook for10 minutes, stirring continuously.

When the cauliflower is tender but firm, stir in the garam masala, ground cumin, coriander and lemon juice and serve.

Supper

Basil & Tomato Scrambled Eggs: 195 calories

2 small eggs

1 tbsp onion, finely chopped

3 fresh basil leaves, finely chopped

4 cherry tomatoes, quartered

2 teaspoons Parmesan-style vegetarian cheese, grated

1 teaspoon butter
Salt & pepper to taste
2 crisp breads

Melt butter in a frying pan over low heat.

Turn heat to medium and sauté the onions for about 1 minute.

Add the eggs, basil, salt & pepper.

Cook for 1 to 2 minutes, stirring constantly to scramble.

Stir in tomatoes and cheese.

Remove from heat when eggs are thoroughly cooked.

Serve with a couple of crisp breads.

Day 14: 495 calories

Breakfast

Baked Spiced Grapefruit: 62 calories

½ medium grapefruit
1 teaspoon clear honey

¼ tsp ground cinnamon

Preheat oven to 190°C/375°F/Gas mark 5

Loosen grapefruit segments with a sharp fruit knife.

Drizzle with honey.

Sprinkle with cinnamon.

Bake for 15 minutes.

Serve hot

Lunch

Mediterranean Vegetable Roast: 91 calories

¼ red pepper, cut in chunks

¼ orange pepper, cut in chunks

½ courgette (zucchini), thickly sliced

½ red onion, sliced

½ tbsp olive oil

½ tsp mixed herbs

Preheat oven to 220ºC, 425ºF, Gas Mark 7.

Put red and orange peppers, courgette slices and onions into a small roasting tin.

Pour on olive oil and mix thoroughly to coat vegetables.

Roast for 30 minutes.

Sprinkle with mixed herbs and serve.

Supper

Spaghetti with Courgette (Zucchini) & Onion: 342 calories

1-cal olive oil spray

½ medium onion, thickly sliced

1 medium courgette, thickly sliced

½ tsp ground black pepper

70g (2½ oz) dry spaghetti

1½ tablespoons Parmesan-style vegetarian cheese

6 large leaves from round lettuce

Cook spaghetti according to instructions on the packet.

Spray frying pan with 8 sprays of 1-cal oil over a medium heat.

Stir-fry onions and courgette slices, seasoned with pepper, for 6-8 minutes until tender.

Remove from heat.

Drain spaghetti, rinse with boiling water and transfer to bowl.

Add vegetables to spaghetti and mix well.

Arrange lettuce leaves on a plate and spoon the mixture onto the bed of leaves.

Sprinkle with cheese and serve.

Day 15: 500 calories

Breakfast

Spiced oranges: 100 calories

2 navel (small) oranges

1 tbsp lemon juice

1 tbsp orange juice

Large pinch ground cinnamon

Stevia to suit your tastebuds

Use a sharp knife to remove the rind and pith from the oranges.

Divide the oranges into segments and arrange in a serving bowl.

Put the lemon juice, orange juice, cinnamon and stevia in a cup and mix thoroughly.

Pour over oranges before eating.

Lunch

Cauliflower Soup: 87 calories

240 ml (8 fl.oz) low sodium vegetable stock

1 tbsp lemon juice

Florets of ½ medium cauliflower

½ tbsp olive oil

1 tbsp spring onion, chopped

Pinch nutmeg

¼ tsp ground black pepper

Boil stock and lemon juice in saucepan.

Reduce heat to medium and add cauliflower.

Cook for approx. 10 minutes until tender.

Warm oil over medium heat in a non-stick frying pan.

Fry spring onion gently for approx. 5 minutes.

Add spring onion to cauliflower and stir well.

Use a hand blender to puree the solids or use a food processor to blend.

Stir in nutmeg and pepper, and serve.

Supper

Mixed Roast Vegetables with Pasta: 313 calories

1 small red pepper cut in chunks

112g (4 oz) fresh mushrooms

1 small onion cut in wedges

1 baby courgette (zucchini) cut in chunks

2 tsp olive oil

¼ teaspoon minced garlic

Sea salt to taste

Ground black pepper to taste

56g (2 oz) pasta

Preheat oven to 220ºC, 425ºF, Gas Mark 7.

Mix mushrooms, onion and courgette with olive oil, garlic and seasoning.

Spread onto a foil-lined oven tray.

Roast for approx. 15 minutes until tender.

Meanwhile, cook pasta according to instructions on package.

Rinse pasta with boiling water and drain.

Transfer to serving bowl and stir in the vegetable mixture.

Serve hot.

Day 16: 499 calories

Breakfast

Cheesy Toasty Breakfast: 99 calories

1 small slice wholemeal bread

28 g (1 oz) cottage cheese

1 tsp cinnamon

1 pineapple ring

Preheat grill to medium heat.

Toast bread on one side.

Spread cottage cheese evenly on untoasted side.

Sprinkle with cinnamon.

Top with pineapple ring.

Grill until cheese begins to brown.
Serve hot.

Lunch

Sweet & Sour Salad: 87 calories

56g (2 oz) cauliflower
3 tbsp fresh parsley, chopped
10 cherry tomatoes
2 g (1 oz) low fat yogurt
30ml (1 fl oz) lemon juice

Cook the cauliflower until tender but firm and leave to cool.
Put the tomatoes and parsley in a bowl.
Add the cauliflower.
Mix together yogurt and lemon.
Spoon onto vegetables and mix well before serving.

Supper

Vegetable Goulash: 313 calories

1-cal olive oil

¼ medium onion, thinly sliced

56g (2 oz) Quorn pieces

1 small green pepper, thinly sliced

½ teaspoon paprika

½ clove garlic, chopped

200g (7 oz) canned chopped tomatoes with juice

½ teaspoon dried oregano

½ teaspoon tomato puree

60ml (2 fl.oz) red wine

Pinch stevia

Sea salt

Ground black pepper

Coat frying pan with 8 sprays olive oil over medium heat.

Fry onion until tender, then add Quorn and green pepper.

Cook for further 5 minutes, stirring continuously until pepper is tender.

Stir in paprika and garlic.

Add tomatoes and juice and stir well.

Mix in oregano and tomato puree and stir in wine.

Bring to boil, reduce heat, cover and simmer for 20 minutes, stirring occasionally.

When liquid is thickened, stir in stevia, salt and pepper.

Serve immediately.

Day 17: 494 calories

Breakfast

Pear and Ginger Smoothie: 190 calories

2 oranges
1 soft, juicy pear
1 tsp clear honey

1 small piece of ginger root (according to taste), finely chopped

Preheat the grill to medium.

Cut the pear in half, removing core and stalk.

Place the halves flesh side up on a baking tray.

Brush with honey.

Heat for about 7 minutes until the flesh is softened and the honey caramelises.

Squeeze the oranges and put the juice in a blender.

Add the pears and blend thoroughly.

Pour into a glass to serve.

Lunch

Coleslaw: 79 calories

28g (1 oz) cabbage, finely shredded

½ medium apple, cored and finely chopped

28g (1 oz) carrot, grated

1 tbsp Dijon mustard

2 tbsp extra light mayonnaise

1 tsp sugar

2 tsp lemon juice

½ tsp cumin

1 sprig parsley

Combine all ingredients except parsley in a bowl and mix thoroughly.

Garnish with parsley.

Supper

Chinese Ginger Vegetables: 225 calories

1-cal olive oil spray

½ inch fresh ginger, peeled & grated

1 small onion, sliced thinly

140g (5 oz) frozen mixed vegetables

84g (3 oz) fresh or frozen French beans, sliced

75ml (2½ fl.oz) water

1 tbsp dark brown sugar

1 tbsp cornflour

2 tbsp soy sauce

2 tbsp malt vinegar

½ tsp ground ginger

Coat large frying pan with 6 sprays of oil over medium heat.

Add ginger, fry for 1 minute.

Remove from pan and drain on piece of kitchen towelling and place to one side.

Place vegetables and water in the frying pan.

Cover, and cook for 5 – 6 minutes until vegetables are tender.

In a bowl, combine sugar, cornflour, soy sauce, malt vinegar and ground ginger.

Add this mix to the vegetables in the frying pan and simmer, whilst stirring, for 1 minute until liquid thickens.

Stir in the grated ginger.

Cook for a further two minutes before serving.

Day 18: 492 calories

Breakfast

Cucumber, Mint & Orange Refresher: 105 calories

½ small cucumber
1 tbsp fresh mint leaves
100ml (3½) fl.oz apple juice
10 ml (3½) freshly squeezed orange juice

Peel and cut cucumber into chunks.

Put cucumber and mint into a blender with apple and orange juice.

Whizz thoroughly until smooth.

Pour into a tall glass.

Lunch

Quick Minestrone Soup: 197 calories

2 medium tomatoes
28g 1 oz) dry spaghetti
250ml (8 fl.oz) vegetable stock
28g (1 oz) frozen peas
28g (1 oz) frozen peppers
Sea salt
Ground pepper

Place tomatoes in boiling water for a couple of minutes to loosen skin.

Remove skin and chop tomatoes.

Break spaghetti into small pieces and add to stock.

Boil stock and add tomato chunks.

Simmer gently for 5 minutes and season.

Add frozen vegetables and return to boil.

Simmer for further 2 minutes until vegetables are tender.

Pour into bowl and serve.

Supper

Pasta with Tomato Sauce: 190 calories

28g (1 oz) penne pasta

1-cal olive oil spray

1 clove garlic, crushed

½ small onion, chopped

28g (1 oz) celery, chopped

20g mushrooms, sliced

1 tablespoon grated carrot, grated

1 small basil leaf, finely chopped

¼ tbsp fresh thyme, finely chopped

200g canned, chopped tomatoes

Ground black pepper

Salt

Put a saucepan of lightly salted water to boil for the pasta.

Coat medium saucepan with 8 sprays olive oil.

Sauté garlic, onion, celery and mushrooms for about 5 minutes whilst stirring, until softened.

Add carrot, basil and thyme.

Cook for a further 5 minutes.

Pour in tomatoes with juice and bring to boil.

Reduce heat to low and season with pepper.

Cover and simmer for about 15 minutes, stirring occasionally.

Meanwhile, add pasta to boiling water and cook according to instructions on packet.

Drain pasta, rinse with boiling water and transfer to plate.

Pour mixture over pasta and serve immediately.

Day 19: 493 calories

Breakfast

Fresh Fruit and Vegetable juice: 145 calories

1 apple
½ small lemon, peeled
3 stalks celery
1 large carrot
227g (8 oz) spinach
Crushed ice

Put fruit and vegetables through the juicer
Place crushed ice into glass
Pour juice over and serve

Lunch

Carrot and Cumin Soup: 108 calories

(Delicious hot or cold)

1-calorie olive oil spray
1 clove garlic, crushed
1 baby leek, chopped,
1 tbsp onion, chopped
½ tsp cumin
Pinch cayenne pepper
120ml (4fl.oz) vegetable stock
1 large carrot, chopped
Ground black pepper

Coat a saucepan with 8 sprays of oil and heat gently.

Add garlic, leek and onion and cook for approx 4 minutes until vegetables soften

Turn heat to medium pour in stock and add cumin, cayenne pepper and stock.

Bring to boil and add carrots.

Simmer for 15 minutes or until carrots are tender

Puree mixture in a blender until smooth
Add ground pepper to taste

Supper

Tofu and Quinoa: 240 calories

90ml (3fl. oz) water
Pinch of salt
42g (1½ oz) quinoa
1 tbsp lemon juice
½ tbsp virgin olive oil
½ clove garlic, minced
Pinch of black ground pepper
42g (1½ oz) baked smoked tofu, diced
¼ yellow pepper, diced
2 cherry tomatoes, halved
42g (1½ oz) cucumber, diced
1 tbsp fresh parsley, chopped
1 tbsp fresh mint, chopped

Add quinoa to boiling, salted water.

Reduce to simmer, cover and cook until all water is absorbed (10 -15 minutes).

Spread out quinoa on a baking tray to cool for approx. 10 minutes.

While it is cooling, whisk lemon juice, oil, garlic, salt and pepper.

Add quinoa, tofu, pepper, tomatoes, cucumber, parsley and mint.

Toss well before serving.

Day 20: 500 calories

Breakfast

Spicy Apple and Kiwi Smoothie: 80 calories

1 small Granny Smith apple, cored and sliced

½ kiwi fruit, peeled

1 small celery stalk

42g (1½ oz) parsley leaves

½ tbsp fresh ginger, minced
1 tsp lime juice

Place all ingredients apart from lime juice into juice extractor.

Stir in lime juice, pour into a glass and serve.

Lunch

Yoghurt Waldorf Salad: 233 calories

58g (2 oz) celery sticks, thinly sliced
1 small red eating apple, cored and sliced
14g (½ oz) chopped walnuts,
14g (½ oz) raisins
56g (2 oz) natural low-fat yoghurt
½ tbsp lemon juice
4 leaves from round lettuce
Sea salt & ground black pepper to season

Thoroughly mix yoghurt and lemon juice.
Add salt and pepper.
Stir in celery, apple, walnuts and raisins.
Refrigerate for approximately one hour.
Serve chilled on a bed of lettuce.

Supper

Spiced Lentil Stew: 187 calories

50g lentils
120 ml (4 fl.oz) water
½ small onion, chopped
1 celery stalk, chopped
70g (2½ oz) canned chopped tomatoes
1½ cloves garlic, crushed
Small sprinkle curry powder (to taste)
Sea salt
Ground black pepper

Put lentils in water and bring to boil.

Turn heat to simmer and add onion, celery, tomatoes and garlic.

Cover and simmer for 35 minutes, stirring occasionally and adding more water if required.

Add curry powder, salt and pepper halfway through cooking.

Conclusion

It is my sincere hope that you might have liked all the recipes which have been mentioned in the book and once again thank you for getting this book and experimenting with the recipes.

About The Author

Keith Love is born with the vision to promote *Intermittent fasting* cooking among the masses. The author has written several research papers on the topic. He has served as an instructor promoting various cultural arts in University of San Francisco. He is currently living with his spouse in Texas.

www.ingramcontent.com/pod-product-compliance
Lightning Source LLC
LaVergne TN
LVHW011945070526
838202LV00054B/4806